I0787931

The Six Figure Fit Pro

How Fitness Professionals Can Make More Money in Less Time

By Matt Pack

Copyright © 2019 Matt Pack
All rights reserved.
ISBN: 9781-798160305
Independently Published

Here's What's Inside...

Introduction

Miami, FL
September 2014

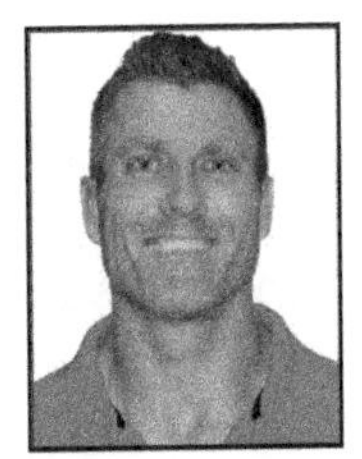

I started out much like all fitness professionals working the typical paradigm of long days and always chasing my next client. After years of trial and error, I realized this wasn't healthy. It wasn't smart and it wasn't why I got into the business in the first place. If I was going to last in this business, a new model was necessary.

I realized that if I wanted to help more people get healthy and fit, then I would have to evolve from using the traditional one-on-one training model. The most important thing to me was how many people I could reach and help – not how many hours I was spending training. I found that the semi-private, small group training model was the best way to shorten my days, increase my earnings and keep the healthy lifestyle I wanted while impacting the most people.

This book is a result of what I learned from years of trial and error. What follows is an interview where I show you my system for creating 6 figures in your training business by working less not more.

Enjoy the book!

I hope this book educates you and helps change your way of thinking about how you run your personal training business and encourages you to take the leap to helping a lot more people fall in love with being healthy.

To Your Success!

Matt Pack

Six Figure Fit Pro!

Susan: Good afternoon. This is Susan Austin and I'm excited to be here today with Matt Pack to discuss how Matt helps fitness trainers make more money in less time. Welcome Matt.

Matt: Thanks for having me Susan. I'm excited.

Susan: You've been on both sides of this coin, haven't you? You've been down the path of working more and making less, if you will. Correct?

Matt: I've spent a lot of time on trial and error and learning from mistakes and fine tuning my business plan, but ultimately I work a lot less than I used to and I'm enjoying my life more as well.

Susan: Why did you want to write this book?

Matt: Well, I feel like I have a good story. I feel like I have the experience to write it. I feel like I've lived it. I've been in the same shoes as a lot of other fitness professionals out there. I know the struggle. I know the day to day grind which can be grueling. I've been in this industry since 1998 figuring out what works and what doesn't and with small group training I've officially found my calling. The goal is to change lives, increasing the health of people but without sacrificing your own. The typical trainer paradigm is a very long day. It usually starts at 5am, and doesn't end until 7 or 8 at night. It can be off and on throughout the whole day, but it's pretty much a non-stop grind. It's hard to find time to get in your own workout. It's hard to get quality sleep and eat healthy when you are running around like that. If you're not the best version of yourself, how can you help someone else on theirs? How can you be a model to your clients when your life is a constant grind? It's so important to not only talk the talk but more importantly to walk the walk. It's a must to practice what you preach.

Susan: Why is the day so long for a personal trainer?

Matt: We don't get paid a salary, and our day is broken up. The prime time hours for trainers are from 5 to 9am. Then there are obviously off peak hours where you could pick up house moms and athletes and stragglers in the gym, maybe people that are retired or maybe older, somebody to fill up the off peak 10 to 4 time slots. However we don't have a 9 to 5 steady clientele, but we strive to get that, and if you're good, you can achieve that 9 to 5 or 5am to 5pm, but at what expense, you'll die! Usually, the 5am, 6am are very popular and then, the 7am and 8am before people go to work. Then after that, it's usually dead. Like I said, you can fill in those time slots with off peak house moms, business owners, boomers, or athletes. It can be long simply because you're trying to make money. You're trying to make it a career. You're trying to make it your livelihood, and you don't really have a choice, you take what's offered to you most of the time.

Susan: They have to work these long 12-15 hour days which goes against what they stand for which is being in peak health and shape?

Matt: Exactly. I've seen unhealthy trainers. I've seen overweight trainers. I've seen sick trainers, sleep deprived trainers, stressed out trainers. You can't practice what you preach if you're not taking care of yourself. It's about time that trainers learn how to work smarter and I'm confident what I outline in this book is the future of the fitness industry. It's different yes, but how is what you're doing now working for you? Would you like to make more money while working less hours? Have more time for your family or your own workouts? Be more rested, attentive and passionate for your clients? Of course you do. If you're like me, you're in this to change lives and help as many people as you can. This is the most efficient way to do just that and it's just the smarter way to go about running your training business. It's a new way of fitness coaching, and it's about quality over quantity, and it's training smarter, not longer.

Why Don't More Fitness Professionals Have Six Figure Practices?

Susan: Why do trainers struggle with having six figure practices?

Matt: There are only so many 6am sessions in the day. There are only so many 6pm sessions in the day, and those are popular sessions; the 5, 6, 7 and 8am are very popular. Then, you have the after work crew: the 6, 7 and 8pm slots. You have to wake up early, and you have to stay late because that's where the demand is. That's just how it is. If the average personal trainer is charging $60 per session or $60 per hour, you can do the math.

That's a decent day at $60 an hour but if you think about it, there is still more time in the day. You're busy in the beginning and the end, but there is a lot of the day that's downtime for the trainers. Obviously, you want to try to maximize the day. If you're good and you hustle, you can do alright, but there is a better way to make a great living being a personal trainer. The goal should be for trainers to help as many people as possible in the same time period, and you can only help so many people get in shape in the one-on-one model. I love to help people in the small group model simply because I help more people all at one time. Instead of helping one person per hour, I'm able to help 8 people per hour.

If you look at the volume of people you can help in a group vs. a private one-on-one, there is no comparison. I want to change the mindset of the trainer to stop thinking about how much money you can make per hour and start thinking about how many people you can help on a monthly basis. I really don't care if I have 2 people show up for a session. Well, I actually do, but I'm not stressed because I have 125 people at Primal Fit Miami and they're paying me on a monthly basis. Everyone pays me up front for the month. They pay for a certain amount of sessions per month that they must use. It's not about how much money I make per hour anymore. It's about how many people per month I can help. That's the hard concept for the one-on-one trainer to wrap there head around. We are so used to charging by the hour. It's all we know.

Susan: The one-on-one model is an old school model where they are trading time for dollars.

Matt: It is.

Susan: The one-on-one training model is what leads to trainer burn out. They are working these long hours, and so they are not as healthy as they want to be because it becomes a grind after a while.

Matt: The one-on-one personal training has its place. It works well in the rehab or post-rehab setting or it could be an older adult that has special needs. It could be an athlete who has an injury but ultimately, one-on-one training shouldn't be your main source of income. It's funny because clients think they need one-on-one attention; they think they have to have this one-on-one time with their trainer. One-on-one training is expensive; it's a luxury for most people. How many people can afford that 60 or 100 dollar per hour three times a week?

There are not a lot of people in today's economy who can afford it. It's a luxury item that some people like to have. It's a status symbol for some. They like to tell their friends, "I have a personal trainer," or "I have a golf coach," or "I have a masseuse."

Let's take a look at where group training has worked. Karate is a great example. Who got one-on-one training in Karate? No one. Karate has always been taught in groups for eons. Think about yoga and gymnastics; think about swimming. How about team sports coached at the high school and collegiate levels. Strength and conditioning programs for basketball, football, baseball and volleyball are also taught in a group model. Why are we so late to the party?

Rarely will you find an athlete in a one-on-one environment. People think they need this special attention when in fact they don't. Most of the time when you have a one-on-one client that is hesitant to go to a small group and they do it anyway, they regret not doing it sooner simply because of the interaction between friends. The interaction between peers is huge in groups. Developing friendships and also the competitive nature of being in a group, the accountability coming from their peers is fun; it's invigorating; it's inspiring; it pulls the best out of you. Having others in the room working towards a similar goal changes everything! It's not just the trainer or coach holding them accountable. It's the whole group. Ultimately what happens is that the clients you're working with get a better result. Isn't that the goal?

How to Get Better Results with
Your Clients...

Susan: Why would they get a better result in group training?

Matt: They get pushed harder. They see what Jane is doing next to them. They see John pushing Dave. They see what they're capable of by seeing what their peers and their neighbors are doing and how hard they are working. It brings something out of them which can't happen in a one-on-one setting. It can be easy to take a break. It's easier to quit or not give 100% because it's just you pushing them. When you see what others are doing, they're going to bring the best out of you. And you know what, ultimately, what it comes down to, is that it's fun. It's just more fun and when exercise becomes fun, it becomes more consistent.

When exercise is more consistent, then you get a better result. It's as simple as that. If I could increase the playfulness and increase the amount of fun someone is having, they show up more, their retention is better, and then they get a better result. When they get a better result, their friends see the results. When their friends see the results, they come to the gym too. Ultimately, you have a better chance of creating a walking billboard for yourself, and the more walking billboards you have walking around your particular area, the more income is going to come into your business.

Susan: I love it. I have worked with the one-on-one personal trainer, and sometimes you have an off day. Maybe you're fighting an infection, or you're low energy that day for some reason, and the thought of going to face that trainer one-on-one is daunting. But when it's a group like you said, you dig deeper and find a way to get there because you don't want to let the group down, but if it's just me and the trainer, I'll probably send a text canceling.

Matt: In the fitness industry whether it would be a diet that you're embarking on in January or any fitness program, any good coach would tell you that you need a good support system to help you on your journey. Whether it would be a supportive spouse at home or whether it would be a girlfriend or a work out partner. By working in a group setting, you become a team. You make friends. You want others to succeed, too. The accountability factor coming from your peers, either friends or your husband or your work out partner, helps you stay focused on bad days. There are days that you don't feel like working out.

If you're running with your friend, now you have a reason to get your butt out of bed, too. It all comes down to helping you stay accountable to whatever your goal is and making it more fun. If a small group can do this, why not? Training in general or fitness coaching or hiring a fitness coach is a luxury item. It is expensive. Depending on the area that you live, it's going to be anywhere from $60 to $150 per hour. The one-on-one personal training model is very limited; you can only reach a certain amount of people with that model because of the price.

You don't want to lower your rate one-on-one; you want to lower your rate and add a friend or add that small group model. If you're charging $80 per hour, why not drop it down to $60, and train Jane with Jack. Now, you have Jack and Jane being charged $60 a session which is a good deal because they know you used to charge $80. Now, instead of making $80 an hour, you're making $120. Let's say, Jane brings in her friend, Cindy, with you and Jack. "Okay, well fantastic." Now, I'll bring my rate down to $50 per hour with you guys since you all are training together. Let's do that math.

Now, you've got 3 people training with you at $150 per hour. Those 3 people are ecstatic because they're saving money. Now, you made it affordable to more people and you're making more money per hour. In the one-on-one training model, you hit a ceiling. You can only make so much in a day simply because there is only a certain amount of time you can meet with clients. There is only one 6am and one 7am hour slot but now, this model allows you to see 3, 4, 5, 6, 7, 8 people at 6am and it allows you to break through that ceiling. It's an imaginary ceiling that was preventing you from helping more people and increasing your income.

Susan: I love it. This new model is so fabulous because now, if you get the 4 people in a group, 50 bucks an hour or even 40, you're making close to 200 bucks an hour. If one person doesn't show, I would imagine if your 7:00 doesn't show and it's a one-on-one, you don't get paid that hour. Here if one person doesn't show up, you're still going to make way more money per hour than you're making with the one-on-one model. This is a great model, Matt.

Matt: There are definitely some challenges though. If you're not doing semi-private or small group this program presents challenges, sure. There are some coaching challenges, absolutely, but I'm going to show people how to get it done and how to do it easily in my coaching course. It can be done and it should be done. You're going to have to get outside your comfort zone. We tell our clients this all the time. You have to get comfortable being uncomfortable. That's the only way change happens and it's not only in the fitness world.

Insanity - doing the same thing over and over again and expecting different results.
~Albert Einstein

Whatever your goal, find someone ultra-successful and take them to lunch. Get them to tell you everything they've done in order to achieve that particular goal. How bad do you actually want what they have? Are you really ready to do what it takes? Sacrifice what they have? Are you ready to get outside your comfort zone? If so, apply EVERYTHING this person has done to achieve what they have achieved.

It's the same thing at body composition. If I see somebody that's lean and has the body that you want to achieve, well, I'm going to ask that person, "Hey, excuse me. What are you doing? You look fantastic. What's your daily activity? What's your daily regimen? What do you eat every meal? I want to look like you." You don't go find somebody that's obese and has the body that you don't want and ask them for advice.

If you want to make a lot of money and help as many people as possible, you find someone that is already doing it. Purchase their product, pay for a consult, pick their brain, you mimic, you imitate. Success leaves clues. Find the most successful people in whatever field they're in and imitate them, apply those habits and tools to your business. Why re-invent the wheel? Follow in the footsteps of those that have already figured it out. Stop trying to reach goals doing things how you "think" it should be done and start doing things how it's been "proven" to be done.

How to Transition Your Clients to Group Training...

Susan: I agree completely. I love what you said, "Success leaves clues." How can they get to where you are Matt?

Matt: The first step is to assess your existing clientele. Hopefully you already have an existing clientele. You're already doing one-on-one, and you're probably exhausted, tired and trying to find a way to make some more money and work less hours. Well, here is how you do it. You approach your client through an email or in person, I suggest actually in person, meet with them and tell them, "I'm changing my business model and here is my goal in the coming year." You may give a date on it. I'm going to start this July 1st of 2014, or maybe even better, January 1, 2015. Whatever you do, pick a date and say, "This is going to be my new business model. Here is why I'm doing it." You explain to them that you want to help more people, and you want to make your services more accessible to others by making it more affordable.

You might have to start this off with 2 people in a semi-private model first and that's a totally great place to start. Instead of charging your usual rate of $80 for one-on-one, you'll charge $60 per person for two people or "semi-private." That's how you start this process. You would double up people in the 6am, 7am, 8am and 9am "prime-time" slots. Then start with your other "prime time" slots like 6pm, 7pm and possibly 8pm. The goal should be to get two people per hour in all of your "prime time" slots. Let's start small with semi-private, make it more affordable for them, and give them incentives to come on board. This is the best way to start your new model. After you've established some semi-private doubles, do your best to add a third person to each of those slots. I think you understand where I'm going with this right?

Susan: I love it. It's a way to transition the current model to introduce your clients to the group model without it going from one-on-one directly to ten on one.

Matt: You got it. They think that they need you by yourself. They're actually pretty selfish which makes me laugh! I'll be honest with you, they want you all to themselves, but when you explain the model, you say, "Hey, I really want to take my business to another level this year. It's important that I help more people. My goal in this New Year or my goal going forward is to help more people, and this particular business, this model that I'm in right now is not allowing me to help as many people as I could. This is what I'm doing going forward. If they don't like it, then you simply refer them to someone else. They can't hold you back from reaching your new goal.

Your goal is to help more people while making more money and working fewer hours. If they trust you and know that they are receiving the same service for less money and will get a better result, I'm confident they will be all over it. You must over emphasize that this is your new business model and it's in their best interest to be a part of the new system. Who's going to complain about getting a better result in less time while investing less money? Trust in the system. You are a business professional.

Susan: From a client's point of view, that's the benefit that they get. They'll get the community effect. They'll get the inspiration, the motivation, beyond what the trainer can provide. I think from a client point-of-view, I can't imagine that they wouldn't be open to this. It's a win-win for everyone.

Matt: What I like to tell my clients is they're still going to get individualized attention. In fact, they won't even notice the difference. They're going to get all the attention they need just in that semi-private training model. They're not even going to notice the difference because it's just 2 of them. They're still going to get to talk about what they did for the day. They're still going to be able to talk about their diet. They're still going to be able to talk about their off day fitness regimen. There is nothing that's going to change as far as their individualized attention. They're actually going to get more value. They're going to get better results at a cheaper rate.

Susan: I love it. Okay, good. That's a great way for trainers to transition their current clients into the new model. I think new clients would be very attracted to this because now it's affordable for the people who aren't doing the one-on-one training. Now, there is a way where they can start getting results without having to pay a more expensive one on one training rate.

Matt: You got it. A great thing about this, too, is now you have 2 people that you're working with; they're going to get fantastic results. Let's say you do that 8 times a day. Let's say you have 8 hours a day that you're training. You're seeing 2 people in each one of those sessions, that's 16 people per day. That's 16 people that are going to be a walking billboard around your neighborhood, around your gym, versus 8. Now, you have doubled the amount of people that potential clients will see changing. This significantly increases the chances of attaining referrals and receiving more customers which obviously increases the profitability of your training business.

How to Create a "WOW" Experience...

Susan: What's something else they could do to start moving toward the *Six Figure* practice?

Matt: The second step is once you have your semi-private model in place and it's working, you have to create a wow experience. What I mean by that is you have to create this value, this customer service value. It's not just all about the work out. The customer service has to be there. This is one of the things that most trainers fail to recognize. We have to be professional. You have to show up looking good with a uniform on, preferably a collar shirt with a logo on it. Not a t-shirt with trainer written on the back. You must look the part. Clean shaven, hair groomed, teeth brushed, have nice breath and deodorant on; NO cologne. You're not going on a date but you are making a statement, a statement that you take your profession and business seriously.

It's important that you give them a wow experience. It's not just about the training or the work out. It's very important that you put a high standard on how you present yourself and that your customer service skills are on point. I'm going to go real deep on the customer service and some of the tricks that we use at Primal Fit Miami that really create that raving fan. Don't just show up on time; show up 10 minutes early, fully dressed and ready to put on a show. You have to be ON!

You're totally into the client, you're smiling, your personality is on, and you must leave your problems and your troubles and all negativity at home. People don't want to hear your problems or how bad your day has been. It's about them, not you! When you're with your client, they're paying you a premium; you have to create that value so they don't even think twice about what they're paying. The service you're providing is "top notch"; it's not as much about the training session as you might think. That wow experience is crucial. This is a great way to set yourself apart from the competition. Trust me when I say that most trainers out there are over looking this very important step.

Susan: It almost should go without saying, but if you want to have a *Six Figure* business, you have to show up, and you have to look great, and you have to be enthusiastic.

Matt: You have to be on. Susan, I'm not joking with you. You said it, it seems like it's a given, but it seems as though everyone has a trainer story. Susan, you probably have a story about your trainer, your ex-trainer, and most people have seen or heard a story or a have a negative experience that involves something unprofessional a trainer may have done. Whether it was how somebody put them on the treadmill for 20 minutes to warm up while they talked on their cell phone. How somebody was eating during the training session. How the trainer may have done something inappropriate like touching someone the wrong way. How somebody was talking to girls during their session or not paying attention. How somebody didn't show up at all, maybe they totally overslept and left them hanging. In any case, most of these examples are common sense and it's pretty obvious you can't charge a premium rate and run a successful business doing things like that.

As Fit "Pros" we must hold ourselves to the highest of standards as we are on the front line of defense. What we say, how we carry ourselves and how we influence our clients or members can seriously affect the outcome of their health in a very positive way. Movement and diet are like medicine and we have the power to PREVENT sickness and illness with our recommendations. Think about that for a moment. Maybe you'll take your job a little more seriously knowing the power that you possess. Maybe you'll keep up with your continuing education by seeking the best to learn from. Maybe you'll work on your weaknesses like program design, nutrition, business development and marketing. I just want you to understand that in order for us to be taken seriously and get the respect that we actually deserve, we have to act as such.

I challenge you to step up your game and strive to become a FIT PROFESSIONAL not just a "personal trainer". I honestly believe if you realize just how important you are, then maybe you'll act and dress the part. Let's change the perception of the personal trainer. Let's prove to the world that we are as important, if not more important than medical professionals as we PREVENT sickness and disease from occurring in the first place. Let's prove to our society that we are more than just jocks, gym rats and muscle heads. We are business men and women with a passion to change lives.

Don't Focus on Price, Focus on Outcomes...

The 3rd step is to sell your service on outcomes, not price. It's not about the price. It's about what the outcome is going to be. Too many trainers out there are afraid to tell people what their price is because they know that most people are going to question the price. The key to overcoming this objection is to not only show the value of your program but more importantly show that it works. You have to have proof and the proof is in the pictures. Most trainers fail to have proof of what they've done. You must have before and after pictures.

You also must have client testimonials. If you have no evidence that what you're teaching people actually works, you can't demand that high number for your services because people won't believe you. It's a must that on the very first day there are "before" pics taken along with some sort of measurements i.e. body fat, weight and circumference. It's imperative that before you get started with a client you must get those base numbers.

I suggest you ask your clients to write a testimonial or preferably video tape them because anybody can write a testimonial. The best is a video testimonial of your client, telling the camera just how awesome you are and how you changed their life. There is nothing better than a video testimonial with lots of emotion and telling people how you helped, how you've changed them, how you've gotten them back into shape. There is nothing better than that social proof that you can show people to prove what you're doing actually works. That's how you sell on outcome, not on price. Once you have plenty of social proof, price will start to become a non-issue.

At the end of the day, RESULTS are what matter the most. Here is my proof, here is my wall of fame in my gym, and here is my booklet of testimonials from everybody that I've changed. Here is my website showing everybody that I've helped change. Money just doesn't matter as much when they can visually see the value. If they know what you're capable of and what you've done and what you do on a regular basis, the investment won't matter as much, I guarantee it.

How to Use Systems to Automate Your Business...

This is a big one. We have a lot of systems at Primal Fit Miami, so I'm not going to give you the whole thing right now, but the main system that needs to be implemented for any personal trainer business is EFT (Electronic Fund Transfer) or running credit cards. You need a credit card system in place immediately, because I know a lot of trainers out there, I did it myself, are carrying around checks in their pocket, and they're unorganized with their money. By utilizing EFT, the money that they owe you for the month will be automatically put in your bank account. Implementing the EFT system will also prevent people from forgetting their checks. It happens and it stinks. For some reason it slips people's minds that what you do is a service. They won't forget their money when they go to Starbucks or to the grocery store but for you, oops! Having a system in place like this will show that you're a real business and you'll find that clients and prospective clients will begin to treat you with a new found respect. The client will love you too. There's no need to have to remember bringing that check in and more importantly you can stop chasing checks every month. Chasing checks makes you look unorganized, and it also makes you look unprofessional.

Susan: It shouldn't be that if the client flakes out on you, the trainer, that you guys lose money, that's not the way it works in the world any longer. Your time is valuable.

Matt: In the personal training industry because it is so personal and because we're so unprofessional and non-businesslike, people do take advantage of us. It happens a lot where people say, "Oh, hey Matt. I'm so sorry. I forgot your check. Can I bring it next Tuesday? Matt, I forgot my wallet. Do you mind if I pay you tomorrow?" We sometimes get taken advantage of, and we let that happen. The best way to prevent this from happening is to not allow for any type of guessing. Everything should be in the contract.

Susan: You do have a contract right?

Matt: I suggest that you get everyone on a long term contract at least 6 months but I prefer 12 months. The clients get charged every month, for the length of commitment. The sessions don't roll over. There needs to be rules that the client knows, and they need to be in a contract. You should have a contract with your client knowing everything, including length of commitment, sessions per month and what credit card they will be paying with. Is there a cancellation policy? Some rules and regulations vary from state to state but your prices, commitment and EFT information are a must.

Contracts are a must but I know trainers are reluctant. Just be re-assured that for 6 or 12 months, you're going to get paid the same every month versus the stress of wondering if you're going to have a cancellation. It's important to have people on a commitment, and then you have a good merchant account system with low interest rate on those credit cards that you can rely on, that every month on the 1st or the 15th, you're going to get paid. If the client doesn't show up, they still get charged.

Susan: Very good. I love it, and that goes back to them being more professional. Having a contract makes this more of a transformation rather than a transaction. It shows you're just as committed to the client's success and hopefully, possibly, sometimes even more committed. This emphasizes, "We're serious about this. We take your health and your fitness very seriously."

Matt: Right and you're running a business, and if you're not willing to agree, then you can go somewhere else, and I think that's good business practice. Most people would do that, and I think another thing you brought up is that a lot of people can get flaky or sometimes money can be an issue. Maybe they have too many bills coming in that month and then the first person to go is your personal trainer, no doubt about it. How do you prevent that from happening? Well, you create a raving fan. You put so much value on your personal training services and what you give them, on the services you provide, that the last thing on the list is getting rid of the trainer. You want to create such a value to your client that they're going to say, "You know what, instead of getting my hair done twice a month, I'm only going to get it done once a month."

Instead of going out to eat every single weekend, they're going to only go out two times a week or two times a month, once a weekend or two times out of the month. It's not going to be you that is sacrificed. Having a personal trainer is a luxury for sure, but if you can get extra-ordinary results, a wow experience and create a raving fan, I guarantee you that you could be a mainstay in your client's budget not for months but for years.

How to Get Extra-Ordinary Results with Proven Programming...

Susan: Number 5, get extraordinary results with proven programming. What does that mean?

Matt: It means you have to have a training philosophy that gets results. This is something that is lacking in the fitness industry simply because most people are doing what they learn out of a body building magazine. However your programming needs to be repeatable and it needs to be able to move into that semi-private group training model because the one-on-one training is a little bit different than semi-private. You have to know how to program it properly. That's something that I'm going to show you in the Six Figure Fit Pro blueprint. That's the CORE of the program!

I'm going to teach you how to program these semi-private small group sessions to most effectively get the most bang for your client's buck. You will also learn how to create a fun environment, keep injury rates low, and most importantly get great results while creating those walking billboards that are so crucial to bringing potential clients into your facility to increase your revenue. It's very important that whatever philosophy you have, it's repeatable and gets great results. I'm going to teach you our way. It's repeatable and I'm confident it will work for you as well.

Susan: Why can semi-private or small group training be more of a challenge?

Matt: You might have two people with two different exercise levels. You might have one person with a knee injury and one person with a shoulder injury. You have two people with two different goals. It's very important to obtain health history and have each client go through the appropriate assessment process. It's important to know what the goal of each person is and what their history is. You can modify and scale workouts according to your client's level and health history. That's the beauty of this; being able to cater to different exercise levels in the same session. There is a "method to the madness" when it comes to training a group but I'll break it down for you easily in the coaching program. In this *Six Figure Fit Pro Model*, I teach you how to do it all.

Susan: You don't necessarily have to have a group of people who are all at the same level to do this group. You're saying you could have someone who is a little further advanced and someone that's maybe just getting back into fitness after time off.

Matt: Absolutely. What you don't want to do is overwhelm a novice or beginner or under work an advanced athlete. That's what this is all about. You must cater to different exercise levels as well as those with different health histories. You may even have a group that is for athletes and a group for novices but sometimes that's just not going to happen because friends want to train with friends, and they may be at different levels.

It's important that you have that knowledge, and you're able to recognize that less is more for that person. You don't want to have that person sore for 3 to 4 days. You don't want that person to throw up.

You have to modify the workout according to who is in your group. It's not about the trainer. It's about the client. We're still not losing that personal attention. We're still not losing that personal touch. It's still personal, but it's just done in a semi-private small group setting.

Susan: I love it. That's very interesting that with some modification you can have the advanced and the beginners work in the same group.

Matt: Absolutely. It can be done. Like I said, there is some learning curve for the coach but nothing that can't be smoothed out.

Susan: I would have thought these groups had to be kind of tailored to the same level of fitness to make it effective, an advanced group, beginner group, moderate group but that's not the case at all.

Matt: No, it's not at all. Through the assessment process, you're going to find out what the level of exercise is for each person. Are they novice? Are they intermediate? Are they advanced? Are they de-conditioned? Are they post pregnancy? Are they post rehab? I mean, you're going to find out all of this through the assessment process and through the consultation with that person. You don't want to throw someone in the mix, knowing that they never worked out before, and they have a history of injury. It's important that you find out as much as you can about the person before you even start. There is no reason why there can't be different exercise levels and people that have limitations or injuries in the same group. The training session would just have to be modified, exercises regressed or scaled back.

The Six Figure Fit Pro Works for All Personal Trainers...

Susan: Is there any trainer for whom your group training model wouldn't work?

Matt: I think it would work for anyone that takes action. If you want to continue to do one-on-one and you're happy and content with your income, then by all means. This book is for people that are tired and are burned out and have hit a financial ceiling. If you'd like to make more money helping more people, then switching over your business model is a no brainer. There are only so many hours in the day. You must maximize them! It's about finding financial freedom, Susan. It's about creating the life that you want. You don't have to let the business dictate your life; you create your own business model.

Susan: I love that you'll be able to reach a lot more people this way. This is a way for the trainers to reach a lot more people, and they then share their results with more people and so on.

Matt: Exactly. Like I said if you have 4 people per session, 8 hours a day or even 3 people per session 8 hours a day, then that's 24 people you're reaching a day. That's just on one day. What about tomorrow? What about Tuesday and Wednesday, and Thursday and Friday? If you have 20 clients right now and you put 2 people in each session, you're going to get 40 clients. That's 40 clients you're helping versus 20. You're making more money. You're helping more people, and you have more people out there talking about how awesome you are which brings in even more people that you could help. Ultimately, all the way around, it's just a more efficient business model.

Here's How to Get Started Becoming a Six Figure Fit Pro...

Susan: I agree. What can they do to go to the next step with you?

Matt: I'm excited to offer a coaching program which goes through every bit of this. It shows trainers how to transition from the one-on-one to semi-private, small group model. It covers customer service and how to create those systems we talked about. It covers how to create a wow experience for your clients to bring in more qualified referrals and leads. We cover how to set prices and how to create the training systems and how to write programs for the small group semi-private model. I take all the guessing out of it. I have a proven model. I've been where they are and I've done it. I've created a $30,000 a month gross income in a 1,400 square foot training space and you can do the same.

Susan: I love it. How can they get in touch with you?

Matt: They can email me at: info@thesixfigurefitpro.com or they can go to my website, www.thesixfigurefitpro.com.

Here Is How to Make More Money in Less Time...

You already know to help clients get fit and get the results they want. The confusing part is not knowing how to do it without getting burned out spending all day in the gym.

That's where I come in. I help trainers just like you build 6 figure personal trainer business while working less, yet reaching more people in the process.

Step 1: Join our coaching program were we share with you the exact steps to transition from one on one training to helping 5x or even 10x the amount of people you do now.

Step 2: We coach you and mentor you to transform your training business so you are making more and working less.

Step 3: We take you by the hand and walk you step by step through the process.

Most trainers think it takes hours and hours of working one on one with clients to build a successful training business.

Now you can make 6 figures, work less and have fun doing it.

If you'd like me to help, just send an email to: info@thesixfigurefitpro.com and I'll take it from there.

About the Author

Matt Pack has an exercise science background and began his fitness career in Washington, D.C. back in 1998. Matt sold his then company in D.C. and started from scratch in Miami where he now owns Primal Fit Miami, a 1400sq/ft group training facility that happens to be one of the most profitable training gyms per sq/ft in the country.

If you'd like to contact Matt he can be reached by email at: info@thesixfigurefitpro.com or you can go to his website, www.thesixfigurefitpro.com.

www.ingramcontent.com/pod-product-compliance
Lightning Source LLC
Chambersburg PA
CBHW050803240726
48654CB00008B/614